Yoga Sex Coupons: Are You Flexible Enough?

I0435459

Katie Stormy Grey

INTRO:

Yoga Sex Coupons may be to difficult for some people to do. I have included some easier ones at the start and they progressively will get a little harder as you go further into the coupons. Try at your own risk. The author, publisher, do not assume any responsibility from anyone getting hurt or property that could be damaged. User assumes all risk from injury or damage. These are for entertainment purposes only.

Now that, that is out of the way I hope you enjoy this book. Be enlightened.

Katie Stormy Grey

Simply Tear Out The Coupons To Redeem

Feet To The Sky
Happy Husband Pose

This pose requires the female to lie on her back on a floor or a bed. She then raises her legs upwards and grabs her feet with her hands pushing her knees in the direction of the floor. This allows everything to be open. The man can then enter her in whichever hole that he wants in this position and allows him a great view. This is a warm up yoga exercise. Have fun tonight!

Backside
of
Coupon

Child Pose

This is another yoga warm up or cool down exercise position that will show the delicate landscape of her back and butt. Have her knee down on her knees sitting back on her heels. Now have her exhale and extend her arms forward in front of her and lay in the yoga position called child's pose. He can then enter her from behind, while she relaxes and enjoys the moment.

Backside
of
Coupon

Downward Facing Dog

This sex position is what you can think of as the V position. Have her on a yoga mat, so she doesn't slip around. She will have her feet shoulder width apart and place hands down on the floor also shoulder width apart. She will be making an upside down V. He can then while standing enter her from behind and enjoy the great view of your butt. Try to focus on your breathing for 5 mintues before giving into the pleasure. Be in the moment.

Backside

of

Coupon

Forward Fold

Have her start in a standing position, the use of a bed or chair can be used if not flexible enough. Have her spread her legs far apart and reach between her legs trying to touch the floor.with her legs straight.If she is flexible enough she can spread the legs wider until her head is touching the floor with the support of her hands. Otherwiseshe can be stretching down to a bed or a chair to be more comrfortable. He can then warm you up by giving you oral in this position or he can enter you from behind.

Backside

of

Coupon

Chakra Kiss Or Intwind Love

Have him be sitting on the bed, chair, yoga matt. She will place herself on top of him and wrap her legs around his torso, while he enters you. Then you both can slowly begin to breath and rock back and forth. In this position when you kiss imagine that you chakra energy is flowing into each other. This is incredibly intamate and a slow build of sexual energy for an intimate night of love making.

Backside
of
Coupon

Reclined Pigeon or Glute Stretch

Have her lie on her back and bring one foot up on other leg. Reach through and grab leg, which will stretch out glute. Have him enter you. You can switch legs if one becomes tired.

Backside
of
Coupon

Lie Back Butterfly Stretch
Reclined Bound Angel

On the bed grab some pillows and place them down near your legs. Now bend both of your knees and touch the bottoms of your feet together resting your knees on the pillows comfortably. Place both hands above your head and bring your hands together. He can then enter you as like in missionary position that leads to a pleasurable night for her.

Backside
of
Coupon

Recline Shoulder Stand

This pose is can be difficult and she may need the edge of a bed to help if it is to difficult. Have her lie down on her back and lift her legs into the air. With the help of her arms se is going to get her bottom off the bed or floor and put her feet up into the air directly below her shoulders. All her weight will now be on her upper back and shoulders wiht her body straight into the air. He can then enter her and this can lead to a mind blowing G spot orgasm if you can hold it long enough.

Backside
of
Coupon

Tree Pose

The normal tree pose you place you foor on your leg, arms in the air holding your balance on one foot. Instead she will be standing and placing her leg on him, while standing on one foot. She can use her hands to hold onto his shoulders. This requires alot of balance and core strength and this is great practice for it. He can then enter her and help by holding onto her leg.

Backside
of
Coupon

Wheel Pose

This requires a good amount of strenght to pull of. Have her lie on her back and bend her knees so her feet are touching the floor. Next she will place her palms near her head and push upwards using her hands and feet. Your back and butt will get off the ground with hands perpendicular to her feet. she can then push up onto her toes. She will be quite open in this position. Her can then enter her standing up. This position really can be difficult, but it feels amazing since you are activating all your muscles, while having an orgasm..

Backside

of

Coupon

Cobra Pose

Have her lie face down on the bed. Spread her legs apart enough that he can sit between them.

Then she will press her plams into the bed and lift her upper body off the bed, while keeping her lower body on the bed. This will stretch her lower spine. He will then enter her from behind in this position.

He can grab your boobs, pull your hair.

Backside
of
Coupon

Wide Leg Straddle

Have him be sitting on a couch.
She needs to stand above him and
get into cow girl possition and enter
him. Then she needs to spread
her legs apart as far as she can
in the splits position.

Bonus: face away from him with
legs spread in split position and
reach for the floor, while he
does all the work. The stretch
and having your head below
your heart will send a rush of
blood to your head during
orgasm. Make sure he is holding
onto your hips tight and you have
your hands ready in case you
begin to slip.

Backside
of
Coupon

www.ingramcontent.com/pod-product-compliance
Lightning Source LLC
Chambersburg PA
CBHW070838310526
45788CB00017B/2029